This journal belongs to:

_____

Five Minutes to a *Healthier* You

A WELLNESS JOURNAL

Hannah Ebelthite

An Hachette UK Company
www.hachette.co.uk

First published in Great Britain in 2019 by Aster, a division of
Octopus Publishing Group Ltd
Carmelite House
50 Victoria Embankment
London EC4Y 0DZ
www.octopusbooks.co.uk

Distributed in the US by
Hachette Book Group
1290 Avenue of the Americas
4th and 5th Floors
New York, NY 10104

Distributed in Canada by
Canadian Manda Group
664 Annette St.
Toronto, Ontario, Canada M6S 2C8

ISBN 978-1-78325-300-5

A CIP catalogue record for this book is available from
the British Library.

Printed and bound in China

10 9 8 7 6 5 4 3 2 1

CONTENTS

WHY JOURNALING IS GOOD FOR YOU

Welcome to *Five Minutes to a Healthier You*, an easy-to-use wellbeing tool that will help you harness your inner health and find peace and vitality every day. Sometimes "becoming more healthy" can seem an insurmountable task, so this journal offers an easy way in.

In every 24-hour period there are 1,440 minutes. Could you commit to investing just five of those minutes to improving your health by practising valuable self-care, creating new positive habits and consolidating and celebrating existing successes? It's not a big ask, but it is a big step toward realizing the healthy, happy individual that you deserve to be.

BABY STEPS...
This journal is all about learning and developing those small-yet-purposeful habits that soon add up to a sense of holistic wellbeing. Our modern, chaotic lifestyles mean it's easy to feel that we're not doing enough to improve our health. People have a tendency to set huge, non-specific goals, such as "do more exercise", "lose weight" or "eat better". But such sweeping changes can feel overwhelming and unachievable.

Smaller tweaks, on the other hand, put goals within your grasp. Each positive change reinforces your commitment to greater health. The sense of achievement that comes from taking a step toward better wellbeing – however small – will spur you on to do more.

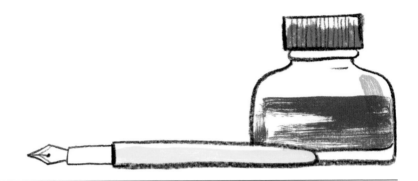

WHY JOURNALING?

Many of the exercises in this book involve writing: these include everything
from writing down key data about your current health, to pinpointing goals,
and stream-of-consciousness, expressive writing. You can use a journal to
look for patterns in past behaviour, to explore obstacles and challenges and
work toward future goals or as a form of daily mindfulness.

And there's mounting evidence in favour of journaling. Studies have
shown that people who record what they eat and drink, in a food diary,
tend to make better food choices and be more successful at losing or
maintaining weight. Athletes and their coaches keep detailed training
logs so that they can plan their development, prevent injury and learn
from the past. Self-appraisal is part of many people's jobs, and students
are actively encouraged to reflect on past work. And, as any teenager who
has scribbled away in a diary can attest, writing down your thoughts and
feelings is a proven way to help relieve stress and anxiety.

It doesn't matter if you don't think of yourself as much of a writer.
No creativity is required – although, by getting into the habit of daily writing
and reflecting, you may discover that you're more creative than you thought.
There are many ways of expressing yourself, whether it's doodling, list-
making, note-taking, mind-mapping or long-form writing. The prompts
in this book will help you to get started in a way that feels right for you.

HOW TO USE THIS JOURNAL

Within these pages you'll find a wide range of tips, exercises, writing prompts and thinking points. They cover all the main pillars of health, from nutrition and fitness, to sleep and mental and social health, to general health and disease prevention. It's up to you how you use this journal – you might like to work through it chronologically, tackling a tip each day. Or you may prefer to dip in at random and try whatever is outlined on the page that falls open. Or perhaps you'll read through it and stop at the suggestions that resonate most with you. (Don't be too discerning, though – sometimes it's the exercises that seem least appealing that can yield the most useful results!)

You might like to keep this journal by your bedside and have your five minutes of "me time" before you go to sleep. Alternatively, it might suit you to have a quiet moment first thing, to invest in your health before the day's demands take hold. Or perhaps lunchtime feels better. There's no right or wrong way – it's your journal, your health and it's up to you. Some of the tips might take just a minute or two to read and ponder. With others you may find your flow and work on them for longer than five minutes – the timeframe is really just a guide.

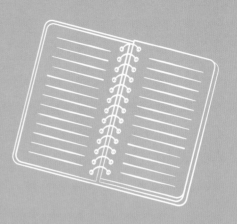

Of course this has not been designed as a finite project. Hopefully, the habit of journaling is one you'll keep up, in one way or another, along with many of the tips and ideas that you encounter in these pages. There will be some exercises that you'll want to return to and make a habit of. Others you can add to your health toolbox, to use in times of need. You can craft a bespoke, self-care plan. And there's something special about moving away from technology and using old-fashioned pen and paper. This is not journaling to be published on a blog, or posted on social media for "likes" and comments. It's for *you*.

The bottom line is that you hold in your hands the means to discover the healthier, happier person who's already within you. The secret to success lies in building healthy habits over time. Starting out with just five minutes a day makes that easy to achieve.

HEALTH CHECK

"The first wealth is health." RALPH WALDO EMERSON

There are times when only a visit to your doctor
will do. But there is also plenty you can do for
yourself, day-to-day, to keep tabs on your
general health. Know your normal and be
ready to take action should anything change.
Knowledge is power – and greater wellbeing.

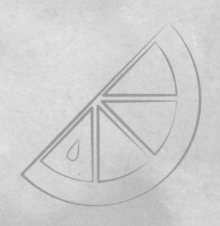

WRITE DOWN YOUR HEALTH WORRIES

What's your biggest health concern? What most worries you about
your own health – now or in the future? It might be a bad habit
you can't seem to break, a fear that you have a genetic predisposition
to a certain condition or an underlying unease about a
symptom you're experiencing. Write about it here.

_____

_____

_____

_____

_____

_____

_____

_____

_____

_____

_____

_____

_____

_____

_____

_____

Think of three practical steps you could take
today, to start alleviating your worry.

1. _____

2. _____

3. _____

KNOW YOUR NUMBERS

How much do you really know about the current state of your health? Our personal health statistics provide important information about our disease risk and often give us an early opportunity to take preventative action. Fill in the blanks opposite, where you can. If you don't know an answer, book an appointment with your doctor or pharmacist to find out. Revisit this page every six months to make sure you're still on track.

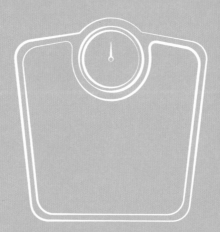

Weight _____

BMI (Body Mass Index) _____

Waist measurement _____

Blood pressure _____

Resting heart rate _____

Total cholesterol _____

LDL ("bad") cholesterol _____

CLEAN BETWEEN YOUR TEETH

Put this journal down, head to the bathroom and floss your teeth – now!

We all *mean* to do this when we brush our teeth, but how many of us really do? Less than a quarter of adults use interdental brushes or floss regularly, yet dentists advise that we all do so, as part of our twice-daily oral-health routine, from the age of 12 upward. It helps prevent gum disease and bad breath, as well as keeping those surfaces in between the teeth clean.

Don't be too aggressive – the idea is to scrape the *sides* of your teeth, from the gums down, to remove food and plaque. Work around your mouth methodically so that you don't miss any surfaces, and don't forget the back of your last teeth.

After you've flossed, brush your teeth using a fluoride toothpaste for two minutes. Then spit, but *don't* rinse – dentists now advise leaving the remaining toothpaste in your mouth, to benefit from the protective effects of the fluoride. Like mouthwash? Choose one that's alcohol-free, but don't use it immediately after brushing. Save it for freshening up, later in the day.

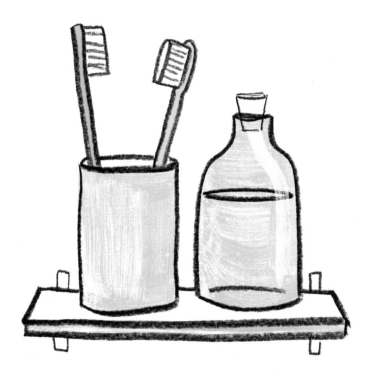

TRACE YOUR FAMILY HEALTH TREE

How much do you really know about your family's health history?
Certain conditions can have hereditary elements, so by being informed
you can better look after yourself and your children in the future.
Make a note of any close relatives who have had a serious condition, and
at what age. If possible, phone your nearest and
dearest to check. Below are some questions you could ask:

- Has a close relative had breast or ovarian cancer?

- Has anyone in the family had high blood pressure,
heart disease or a stroke?

- Do any relatives have high cholesterol?

- What age did my mother go through the menopause?

- Has anyone suffered from recurrent depression?

- What did my grandparents/great-grandparents die of?

- Any other major diseases in the family?

If you're concerned about the impact of your findings
on your own health, speak to your doctor.

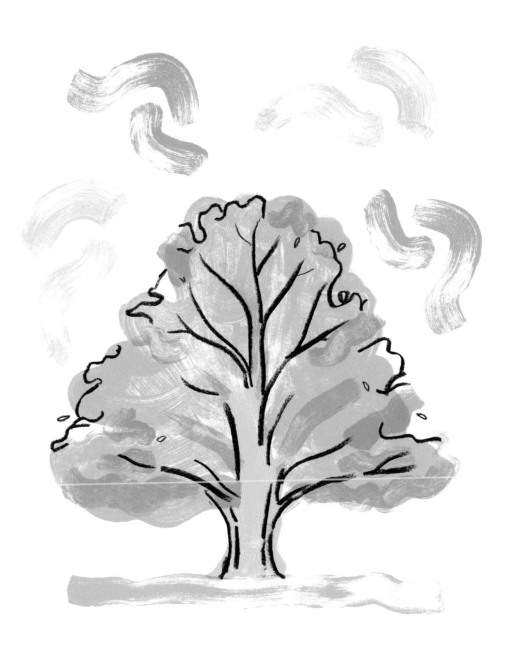

KNOW YOUR OWN NORMAL

Breasts, testicles, moles, general lumps, bumps and marks . . .
It's vitally important to be aware of any changes in the appearance
or feel of your body. But that isn't as easy as it sounds, unless you're
familiar with what's normal for you. Annotate the image opposite to
record body features that may be unusual, but are normal for you.
If they change (breasts over a menstrual cycle, or moles/freckles
in summer, for example), note how.

If there are any new lumps, swellings, marks, rashes or other signs
that you're concerned about – now or in the future – you can also
log them here, along with the date you first noticed them.
And, of course, report them to your doctor.

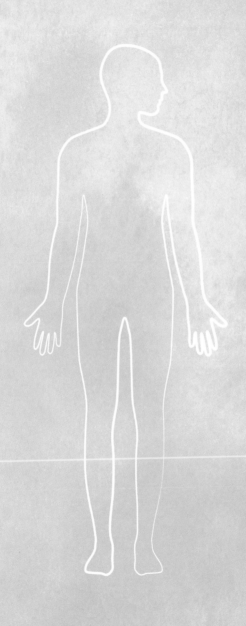

GET UP-TO-DATE WITH ROUTINE APPOINTMENTS

When is your next eye test, dental appointment, hearing test, cervical smear, mammogram or bowel-cancer screening test due? Or, if you're under medical care for certain conditions, when is your next routine check-up or medication review? Don't put it to the back of your mind or put off making an appointment. Spend five minutes investigating, then use the opposite page to record when your last relevant appointments were – and when they'll be due again.

APPOINTMENT	DATE

BOOST YOUR IMMUNITY WITH MASSAGE

It's one of the oldest therapies, common to all conventional and alternative medicine systems. And its effects are holistic – massage is well known to increase all-round feelings of physical and mental wellbeing. As well as boosting blood and lymph circulation, easing sore muscles, relieving back pain and stress, massage has been shown to relieve the side-effects of some cancer treatments.

If you can, book yourself in for a massage – or enlist a friend and offer to give each other a neck and shoulder rub.

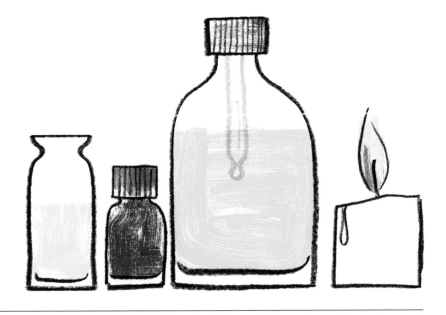

ENJOY

"Happiness doesn't just feel good, it does you good, too. It can even help you live longer." MIRIAM AKHTAR

This chapter looks at your emotional, social and mental health. We'll cultivate kindness, gratitude and happiness. We'll think about self-care, scheduling and technology use. And we'll practise techniques like breathwork, meditation and visualization.

REMEMBER TO SAVOUR

Happiness experts know that one of the keys to contentment is a step on from mindfulness. Yes, it's important to "be" in the present moment, to use all your senses to notice your surroundings: what you can see, hear, smell, touch and taste. But what's also useful is to actively seek out the wonders around you, to find enjoyment in them – to savour, relish, delight and be enthralled – whether it's the people around you, the food in front of you, the bird you can hear singing or the cloud formation above you.

Spend five minutes writing a list of people and things you're grateful for today. Then commit to savouring them – and all the other positive experiences you will encounter today.

PLAN YOUR DAY

If you feel there aren't enough hours in the day – and definitely none left over for you – this exercise will help you to create some.

Think about everything you need to get done tomorrow: places you need to be, jobs to complete, everything from exercise to meals and travel time. Then use the space opposite to schedule your day, from waking to going to bed, with as much detail as possible.

It might seem like an extra task on your to-do list, but this is a technique used by many a business executive to streamline their day, get more done in less time, create headspace and downtime. If you've scheduled one hour to do an online grocery shop between 10 and 11am, you'll stick to it, rather than procrastinating and surfing. You may even get it done sooner, and then you'll have some bonus "me time". Try it for one day and see the benefits.

TIME	TASK	✓

BE YOUR OWN HEALTH INSPIRATION

Use the opposite page to describe in some detail a time in your life when you felt healthy, fit and happy . . .

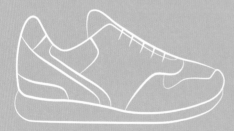

Remember, this is not a celebrity or a social media star that you have described – it's *you*. And it can be you again.

_____

_____

_____

_____

_____

_____

_____

_____

_____

_____

_____

_____

_____

_____

_____

_____

_____

_____

_____

BACK TO WELLBEING SCHOOL

The human brain is happier, younger and more peaceful when it's learning. When was the last time you devoted yourself to learning a new skill? In today's fast-paced society of instant gratification, slowing down – being in the moment and unlocking added neural pathways through learning – is a rare and valuable way of looking after your mental health. And it can provide greater social connections, too, if you want it to.

Try to come up with five different skills or activities you'd like to master. They could be physical, such as a form of dance or sport, or creative, such as pottery, life drawing or playing the piano. Or something more cerebral, like learning a language or getting to grips with a new computer system.

1. _____

2. _____

3. _____

4. _____

5. _____

Choose one skill and research how you can make it happen.

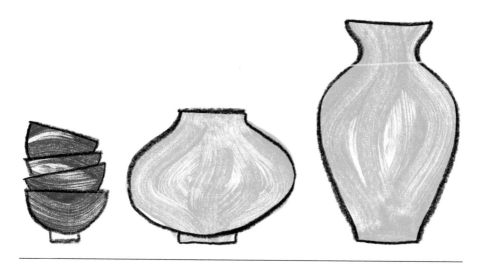

RESTORE
NATURAL ORDER

Go online, or head to the supermarket or garden centre, and treat yourself to a new houseplant. Not only does gazing upon greenery soothe the mind and reduce stress, but indoor plants are known to be air purifiers. They convert the carbon dioxide we breathe out into oxygen and can remove toxins from the air. Given that we spend 90 per cent of our time indoors, where the concentration of some pollutants can be two to five times greater than outdoors, it's more important than ever to become green-fingered.

Both NASA and the UK's Royal Horticultural Society confirm that plants improve indoor air quality by removing volatile organic compounds (VOCs). These are potentially harmful substances, like formaldehyde and benzene, that are released from furnishings and fabrics, paints and household cleaners. Central heating, gas cooking, open fires, log burners and even candles can also contribute to indoor pollution. NASA recommends two plants per 9.3sq m (100sq ft) in your home – the bigger and leafier, the better. Some of the most effective purifiers are spider plants, dragon plants and ferns. Or up your interior-design game with a structural, fashionable plant like a *Monstera deliciosa* (Swiss cheese plant) or *Pilea peperomioides* (Chinese money plant).

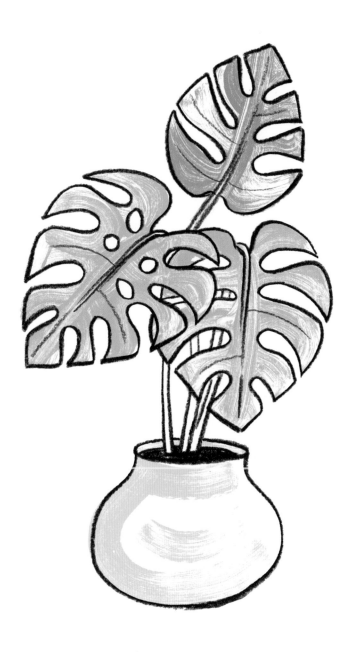

EXERCISE
YOUR BRAIN

Can you solve this puzzle in five minutes?

			8					9
	1	9			5	8	3	
	4	3		1				7
4			1	5				3
		2	7		4		1	
	8			9		6		
	7				6	3		
	3			7			8	
9		4	5					1

NOURISH YOUR SKIN

Find some body lotion or oil and spend five minutes smoothing it over your body, massaging it in and gently relieving tension from your muscles while soothing your skin. Use circular motions and work from your ankles and wrists up your body. Enjoy the scent of the lotion and the feel of it on your skin. Even if you're used to doing this every day after your shower, make this a less practical and more nurturing, mindful time of self-care. This simple, sensual act can increase feelings of wellbeing and self-esteem and put you back in touch with your body.

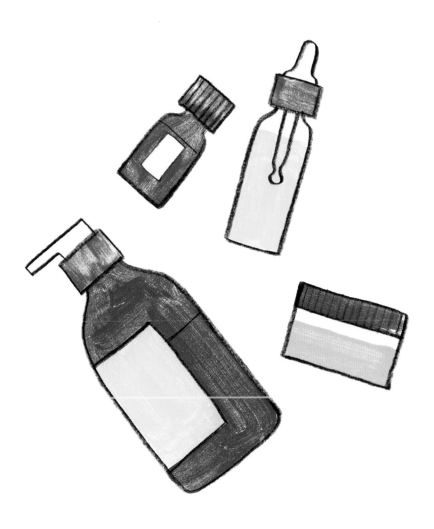

IDENTIFY YOUR "ONE THING"

"Extraordinary things are directly determined by how narrow you can make your focus."

GARY KELLER

It's easy to feel overwhelmed and scattered, if our to-do list has more entries than there are hours in the day. Try writing your list using three colours: one for "must dos", one for "should dos" and one for "would like to dos".

What's the most important thing on your "must-do" list? This is the "One Thing" you need to achieve today. Everything else is just a bonus. Focus on the One Thing first and, once you've completed it, your sense of achievement will fire up the rest of your day.

- _____
- _____
- _____
- _____
- _____
- _____
- _____
- _____
- _____
- _____
- _____
- _____
- _____
- _____
- _____
- _____
- _____
- _____
- _____
- _____

"PIN" THE LIFE YOU WANT

Start work on a mood board that encapsulates all the different elements of a healthy you. This could be online on a platform, or, for greater effect, use a magnetic or cork noticeboard or a large sheet of card – that way you can always keep it within sight

In the centre, put a photograph of yourself that you love. Then position images, quotes, clippings from newspapers and magazines, photos – anything that inspires you to achieve your dream – around your image. Don't think too much and "curate" your mood board. Simply choose items and images that you're drawn to: the natural world, places you'd like to visit, your dream home, a pet you'd love to own – anything you'd like more of in your life.

Your mood board can be a work in progress, so add to it whenever you find something else. But keep it somewhere you'll see it daily, such as your bedroom. The idea is that the images speak to your subconscious mind, giving you a focus for visualization and motivating you to turn your dreams into reality.

PRACTISE LOVING-KINDNESS MEDITATION

"May all beings be happy and secure, may they be happy-minded."

FROM THE *METTA SUTTA*

This popular, contemplative form of meditation focuses on developing feelings of compassion toward others. It comes from the Buddhist tradition called *Metta Bhavana* – cultivating benevolence – but can be practised by anyone interested in fostering love, kindness and empathy.

- Sit comfortably in a quiet place and close your eyes.

- Take a few deep, slow breaths and try to relax.

- Focus on a feeling of inner peace and complete physical and emotional wellness. Feel a sense of love and acceptance for yourself, just as you are. Breathe out any tension and breathe in self-love.

- Silently repeat some of the following phrases to yourself:

"May I be happy"

"May I be safe"

"May I be healthy, peaceful and strong"

"May I give and receive appreciation today".

- Stay with these feelings of self-compassion for a few moments. Then move your focus outward, first to someone you love unconditionally, such as a parent or child. Feel a strong sense of gratitude and repeat the above phrases with them in mind.

- Next take your focus and phrases further out, to other cherished people in your life. Then to wider friends, neighbours, colleagues. You can move on to those you feel neutral or indifferent toward, and then to anyone with whom you are in conflict.

- Finally, send your love out to all beings across the world, focusing on a feeling of connection, empathy and kindness.

BECOME A TWITCHER

The simple pleasure of watching birds in flight or hearing their song can have a surprising effect on your wellbeing. One study found that when the number of birds people saw in an afternoon increased, there was a corresponding decrease in levels of stress, anxiety and depression. Further research suggests that listening to birdsong improves attention span and reduces stress.

Spend five minutes today observing your feathered friends. Sit in the garden, park or on a balcony, even look out of the window. If you don't already do so, you may like to put out some bird food to encourage visitors. Make a note here of the birds you see, what they were doing and how they made you feel.

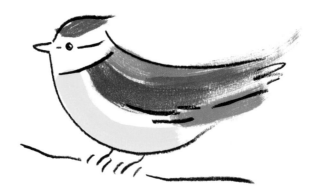

TRY FIVE-COUNT BREATHING

The age-old advice to "take a deep breath" when you're stressed now has science to back it up. You might think of breathing as an automatic process – as, indeed, it is for many animals. But humans are able to choose to alter their breathing pattern. And recent research has shown that breathing at a different pace, or paying close attention to our breathing, alters connectivity in the brain and engages parts normally inaccessible to us Give it a try with this calming breathing exercise:

- Breathe in for a count of five, expanding your belly and then your ribcage. Hold for a count of five.

- Breathe out for a count of five, contracting first your ribcage and then your belly. Hold for a count of five.

- Repeat five times.

1 2 3 4 5

1 2 3 4 5

1 2 3 4 5

SHIFT OUT OF VICTIM THINKING

When we respond to negative situations with thoughts such as "Why is this happening to me?", we're adopting a victim mentality. Much more useful is to think, "Why is this happening *for* me, and what might I learn from it?"

Often we have no control over things that happen in our lives. What we *can* control is our response. Taking the latter attitude – that there's something to be learned from every scenario – is empowering.

Spend a few minutes writing about any resentments that you've felt recently. How can you shift out of victim thinking and look at the situation in a new light?

USE YOUR PHONE INTENTIONALLY, NOT IMPULSIVELY

Are you a slave to your smartphone? Do you find yourself checking texts, emails and social media, or reading the news online, whenever you have a moment to spare. Our constant connectivity is a major source of modern-day stress. It's no surprise people who check their phones frequently experience higher levels of distress during their downtime.

Make sure you're in charge of your phone and not vice versa. Plan three or four times a day when you will check in with your apps and social media. The rest of the time disable mobile data, so you can still receive and make calls and texts, but won't be tempted to surf. Stick to this for at least three days and see how it impacts on your mood.

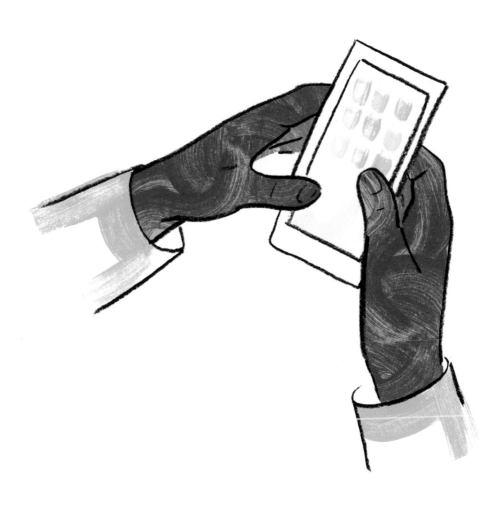

REKINDLE YOUR FRIENDSHIPS

Solitude can be a tonic, but human beings are social animals: we also need to be around other people. Spending time with friends and family has significant mental-health benefits. But these days families may not live close to each other. And social media means we can have hundreds – if not thousands – of connections online, but fewer face-to-face conversations in the real world. It's no wonder loneliness is being dubbed a 21st-century epidemic. How often have you cancelled a social arrangement for a night alone on the sofa, or sent an email instead of meeting someone for a chat?

Use the opposite page to make a list of people you value, whom you would like to speak to and see more often. What's stopping you? Pick three people to call – not text – this week, and make firm plans to meet up with at least one of them.

LOOK TO THE SKY

Next time you're feeling anxious or overwhelmed, lift your head and look up at the sky or ceiling. Studies show that we tend to cast our eyes down when we're sad or scared.

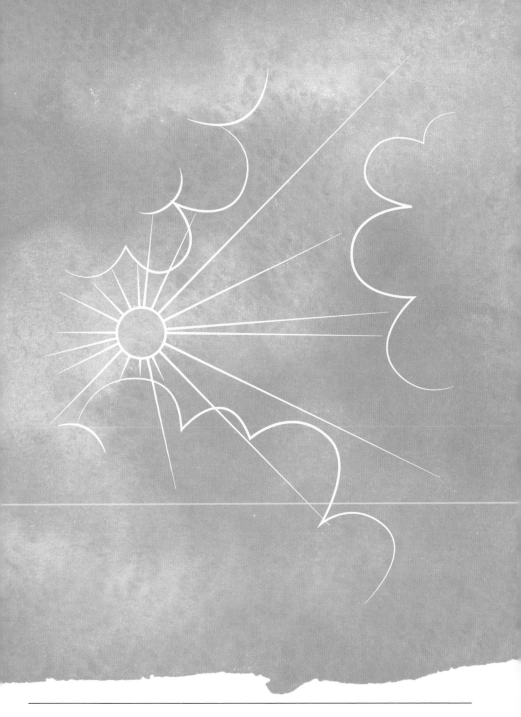

PREDICT YOUR OWN HAPPINESS

Write down how you'd like to see your life looking in five years' time: the very best-case scenario. Research suggests that people who do this regularly are more hopeful about the future than those who keep a diary recording recent events.

Where do you see yourself living in the future? With whom? What are you doing for a living? For fun? How are you feeling? See it, believe it and become it.

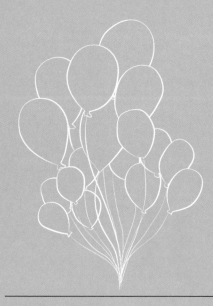

MOVE

"You're in pretty good shape for the shape you are in." DR SEUSS

Who knew five minutes of movement could inject
so much energy – and calm – into your day?
In this chapter we'll learn to celebrate, appreciate
and motivate. We'll learn quick fit tips for lasting
results, break down barriers and find a body balance.

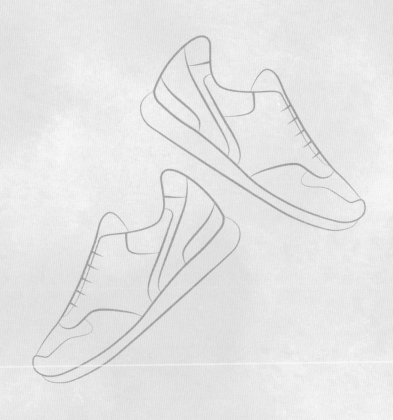

WHAT ARE YOU PHYSICALLY CAPABLE OF?

It's more than you think. A good way to take the focus off how your body looks is to concentrate on how it *feels* and what it can *do*. Take a moment to consider what your body has done for you today, or in recent weeks and months. It doesn't have to be running marathons or scaling mountains, although it's fine to include fitness achievements if you're into them. It doesn't matter if you feel unfit or you're injured – focus on the positives. Jot your thoughts down opposite, in the first person and in the present. Here are some suggestions to get you started:

- I can walk upstairs.

- I can run for the bus.

- I can carry my child.

- I can play a round of golf.

This will shift you into a can-do mindset, where you better appreciate your strengths instead of your weaknesses. Add to this list whenever you notice another element to your physical prowess. You'll soon be surprising yourself by what you can do.

MIRROR, MIRROR

Next time you're getting dressed or undressed, stand in front of a mirror and take a good look at yourself, from head to toe. Find five things that you love about yourself. Write them down opposite and say why you love them. If you find this hard to do, pretend you're not looking at yourself, but at a dear friend, whom you'd only ever view kindly.

Whenever you find your inner critic talking you down, focus on these plus points. For example:

- I love my strong, shapely calves because they can run fast.

- I love my "mum tum" because it tells the story of my children.

- I love my arms – they're strong and hard-working.

- I love my crooked teeth because they give me a cute, quirky smile.

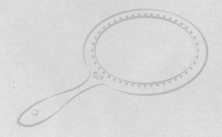

PLAN A MORE ACTIVE DAY

Most of us could do with sitting less and being more active on a daily basis. Research shows that physical inactivity leads to an increased risk of heart disease, diabetes, obesity, cancer, backache, dementia, depression and muscle degeneration.

Use the space opposite to map out your typical day, hour by hour, then look for easy opportunities to fit in more activity. If you have an active job, but tend to laze around at the weekends, plan a weekend day. If you're a weekend exercise warrior, but spend your weekdays desk-bound, then work on your weekday.

Add in every task, journey, every period of downtime. Then think about jobs that you could do in a more active way (pace while making phone calls, use a standing desk); stealthy exercise you could squeeze in (some squats and calf-raises while waiting for the kettle to boil); or some fitness sessions you could create (cycle to work, lunchtime Pilates, power-walk home).

You'll soon notice that all the small injections of activity add up to a more energized, fitter you.

TIME	WHAT I'M DOING	HOW I COULD MAKE IT MORE ACTIVE

WHAT'S YOUR FITNESS MOTIVATION?

Whether you're new to exercise, trying to return to former levels or want to increase your strength and fitness, having a goal to work toward will make you more likely to succeed. It could be losing a certain amount of weight, running a distance you've never covered, lifting a specific weight, learning a different skill or sport or simply fitting in a number of exercise sessions per week.

As well as making your goal Specific, Measureable, Achievable, Realistic and Timely (the SMART concept, popular in business), what really helps is knowing your true motivation. And a good way to get to the heart of this is to keep asking yourself "Why?"

In the space below, write down your current fitness goal.
(e.g. I want to be able to run 5km/3 miles.)

Then ask yourself: why?
(e.g. So I can feel fitter.)

But why?
(e.g. So I can join the rest of my family at parkrun.)

And again, but why?
(e.g. So I can make them proud of me.)

Keep going until you've thought of all the reasons you want to achieve your goal and have found your ultimate motivation. That's what will keep you going when the going gets tough.

_____

_____

_____

_____

_____

_____

_____

_____

_____

_____

_____

_____

KEEP A
TRAINING LOG

Not just for elite athletes, a training log is for anyone and everyone who exercises. It keeps you focused on the benefits of keeping fit, helps you monitor your progress and identify setbacks. It also helps you stick to a workout regime if you schedule sessions in advance.

Start with the week ahead. Write down opposite three times when you're planning to exercise. When the time comes, leave a few minutes after your workout to jot down how you felt before, during and after it. What did you achieve? Did anything feel uncomfortable? What felt good?

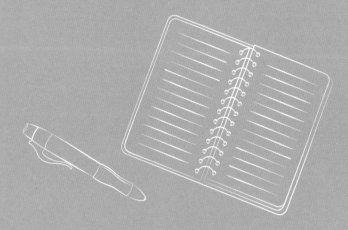

GO HARD, GO EASY

"Intensity is more important than duration. Relative to all sorts of health benefits, it is more time-efficient to exercise hard for a short amount of time than it is to exercise easy for a long amount of time."

MARTIN GIBALA, HIIT PIONEER AND AUTHOR OF
THE ONE-MINUTE WORKOUT

With lack of time cited as the biggest barrier to exercise, it's no surprise that high-intensity interval training, or HIIT, has been *the* fitness phenomenon of the past decade. It consists of multiple short bursts of very intense exercise, interspersed with shorter periods of recovery, and an entire workout can be done and dusted in minutes. Plenty of research supports this method as beneficial for our health, fitness, fat-burning and longevity.

EXAMPLE

- Swipe to the stopwatch on your phone and press start.

- Warm up with 60 seconds of jumping jacks or jogging or marching on the spot.

- Exercise hard for 20 seconds, then recover by taking the intensity right down (marching on the spot, for instance) for 10 seconds.

- Do this eight times, for a total of four minutes.

You can choose any form of exercise that suits you: on a stationary bicycle, treadmill, rebounder, elliptical trainer, even in the pool. Or you can do own-bodyweight exercises, such as high knees, squats, side-to-side jumps, burpees and press-ups. Repeat the same exercise, alternate a pair or make up a mini-circuit – the choice is yours.

FIND YOUR INNER CHILD (OR BOXER)

. . . and get skipping. A skipping rope is one of the best items of fitness equipment to keep handy at home. You'll get a full-body aerobic activity in just five minutes. Skipping mobilizes all your joints, working your arms, legs and core as well as your heart and lungs. And because it's a weight-bearing exercise, it's good for maintaining bone density, too.

If you've not skipped since the school playground, it might take a few tries to regain your confidence and coordination. Start slowly and keep your jumps low. As you get the hang of it, pick up speed and keep to a rhythm and you'll be able to skip for longer. Play around: jumping both feet together, alternating (boxer-style) or hopping. Keep your hands at waist height, elbows close to your sides. Swing from your wrists, not your shoulders, and land on the balls of your feet, keeping the knees soft. Not sure if your rope is the right size for you? Put one foot on the middle and hold the handles up – they should be level with your chest.

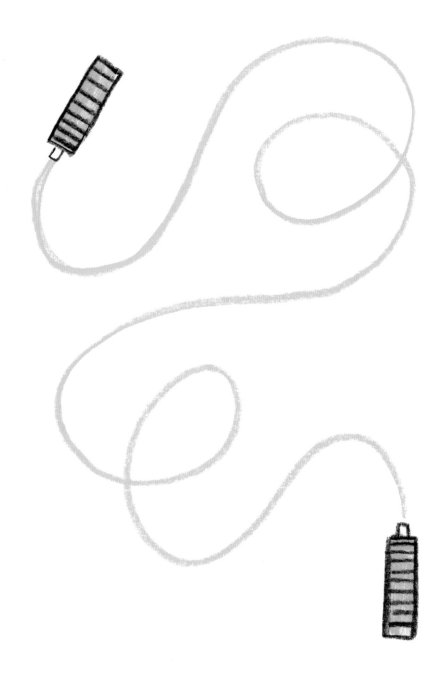

WORK ON YOUR BALANCE

Whenever you brush your teeth, stand on one leg. Change legs after one minute. If that's too hard, rest your fingertips lightly on the edge of the basin to steady yourself. Remove them as it becomes easier. Already easy? Close your eyes.

This develops balance and helps strengthen your core, along with all the small stabilizing muscles around your ankle, knee and hip joints. Tip: draw your pelvic floor up, pull your lower and upper abdominals in toward your spine and clench your buttocks.

You can do this while waiting for the kettle to boil, standing in queues, chatting on the phone, anywhere at all . . .

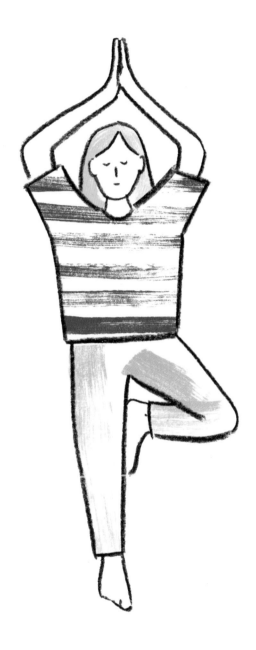

WHAT ARE YOUR FITNESS BARRIERS?

Brainstorm all the factors that you believe are keeping you
from exercise, or stopping you from being as fit as you could be.
Write down whatever comes to mind.

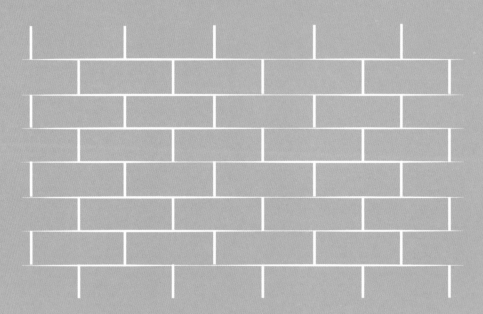

_____

_____

_____

_____

_____

_____

_____

_____

_____

_____

_____

_____

_____

_____

_____

_____

_____

Now pick three and think of one way of
overcoming each barrier.

1. _____

2. _____

3. _____

PACK A KIT BAG

If lack of time or motivation is an issue for you, make "Be prepared" your new fitness motto. If you want to go for a run tomorrow, get your kit ready and laid out the night before. If it's chilly, put it on the radiator to warm. When you get up, commit to the run by putting on your active-wear straight away – you're less likely to get side-tracked during the day.

If you favour the gym, pool or classes, make up a sports bag that's always ready to go. Put in a towel, miniature toiletries, a water bottle, a healthy post-workout snack bar, your trainers and a clean set of gym or swim clothes. Replenish it after every workout and you're good to go.

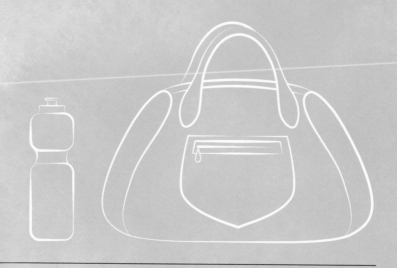

GO FOR A RUN

A five-minute run might not seem worth it, but research suggests it is. One study found that runners were 30 per cent less likely to die over 15 years than non-runners, and 45 per cent less likely to die of a heart attack or stroke. But there was no difference between those who ran for less than an hour a week and those running for three hours or more – proving that less is, sometimes, more[1]. Even running at a slow pace (less than 9.6kph/6mph) was effective and counts as vigorous-intensity activity – getting your heart rate up on a regular basis, through running, improves blood pressure, cholesterol, heart, lung and brain function, and a whole host of other measures.

You could add a five-minute jogging warm-up before a fitness class or gym session, fit it in during a play in the park with the kids or dog, at the end of a walk or to run an errand . . . get creative and get moving.

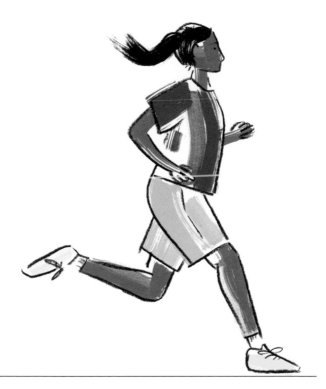

LIE DOWN

It doesn't sound much like fitness, but according to teachers of the Alexander Technique – a system of re-education of the postural mechanism, dating back more than 100 years – lying down can have huge body benefits.

Once a day lie on your back on a firm surface – the floor rather than a bed or sofa. Have your knees up, feet flat, hands resting on your torso. Put a couple of paperbacks or a yoga block under your head to keep your spine aligned. Now relax for five minutes – longer if you have time.

Lying like this releases your spine and neck and all the muscles surrounding them. Gravity enables your shoulders to drop and your chest to open. The pockets of fluid in between your vertebrae that are crushed all day, when standing, get a chance to plump up and rehydrate, lengthening your spine. When you get up you'll be 0.6cm (¼ in) taller.

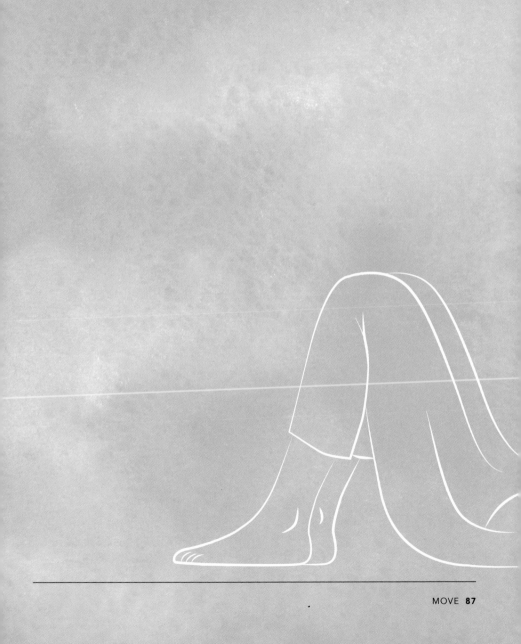

MAKE NATURE
YOUR GYM

It's long been reported that taking exercise outdoors, in nature,
decreases the risk of mental illness and increases feelings of wellbeing.
A large analysis looking at a diverse range of activities, from walking and
gardening to horse-riding and fishing, found that people of all ages and
social groups saw improved mental and physical health. And while all
natural environments offered benefits, green areas with water were
the most conducive to good results.

When it came to the dose? Five minutes' green exercise produced
the largest positive effect on self-esteem.

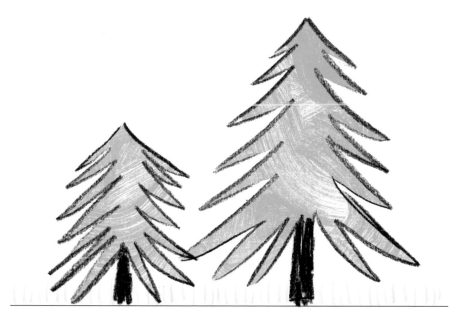

GO BACK TO BELLY BASICS

Forget endless crunches or holding a plank ad infinitum if you want a flatter tummy. Real strength and tone come from an engaged core and an active pelvic floor.

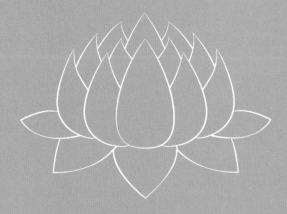

ENGAGE YOUR CORE

You can do this exercise any time, anywhere, whether you're standing, sitting or even lying down.

- As you exhale, draw your belly button back toward your spine. At the same time, draw up through your pelvic floor – think about contracting the muscles you'd use to stop peeing mid-flow.

- Inhale and release.

- Do six to eight slow, controlled movements, followed by six to eight faster pulses.

The more you practise, the more you'll understand what an active core feels like. Keeping the abs and pelvic floor engaged in this way should be the foundation of any other abdominal exercise and, indeed, any form of exercise you do.

DANCE YOURSELF DIZZY

"Nobody cares if you can't dance well, just get up and dance."

MARTHA GRAHAM, DANCER AND CHOREOGRAPHER

The perfect antidote to a sofa- or desk-bound day: put on your
favourite upbeat piece of music and lose yourself in it. Dance, leap,
jump around, do the twist, head-bang . . . whatever feels good.
If you're feeling sociable, get everyone around you involved.
If you're feeling shy, close the curtains!

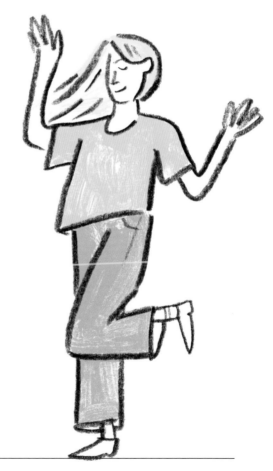

NOURISH

'Tell me what you eat and I will tell you what you are'

JEAN ANTHELME BRILLAT-SAVARIN

Work out what you're really eating, how it makes you feel, then make a few simple adjustments to feel better. From mindful eating to food swaps, recipe ideas and table manners, this chapter is packed with quick and nourishing healthy-eating hacks.

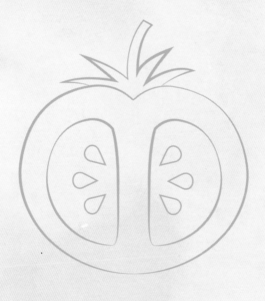

KEEP A FOOD DIARY

Do you *really* know what you're eating? When you lead a busy life you can lose track of what you're consuming – or not consuming – during the average day. Studies have shown that people who keep a daily food diary lose twice as much weight as those who don't. But it's not just about weight loss. It could be that you're skipping meals, not eating enough. A food diary is a brilliant way of keeping track.

For today, make a note of every drop and morsel that passes your lips: the time, what you ate and drank (including the brands) and how much.

At the end of the day you can get an accurate picture of your diet. Do this every time you need to check in on your eating habits, to make sure they're balanced, varied and nutritious. Some questions to ask:

- How many meals did I have today?

- What did I drink, and when?

- How many snacks did I have?

- Did I have some protein and carbohydrate at every meal?

- How much of the food I ate was processed?

- How many portions of fruit and veg did I manage?

WHEN	WHAT	AMOUNT

BE YOUR OWN
DIET DETECTIVE

If you're experiencing particular physical or emotional health issues,
it's worth keeping up your food diary for a week or more to look for
patterns. Is that mid-afternoon energy slump worse if you have wheat
for lunch, say? Does your acne flare up when your dairy consumption
is high? Or perhaps those digestive issues can be explained
by a surprising ingredient?

Revisit your food diary but this time note how you felt before and after
each meal or snack, either physically or emotionally. For example,
you may have felt irritable or tired, or had flare-ups of conditions
like eczema or Irritable Bowel Syndrome.

WHEN	WHAT	NOTES
9am	Large coffee and croissant	Tired and hungry before; more alert after, but still hungry
11am	Tea and two cookies	Needed a pick-me-up
		GENERAL NOTES: Stressful, exhausting day

After a week you might start to see patterns that suggest explanations – and solutions – for your health issues. You could take your diary to your doctor, or to a nutritionist or dietician for their advice.

KEEP UP THE GOOD FOOD WORK

It's all too easy to be hard on ourselves when it comes to diet. But the chances are you're doing a lot that's right. Have a think about what you ate and drank yesterday, or over the past week. Note down all the foods you tried or meals you ate that were healthy. Aim for at least five. For instance:

• I always drink at least 1.5l (2½pt) of water daily.

• I have fruit or veg with every meal.

• I no longer have sugar in my tea.

• I cook dinner from scratch three or four times a week.

You see? You're healthier than you think. Remember how good it feels to make these choices. Give yourself credit where it's due, and try to build on them – to feel even better.

EAT THE RAINBOW

This is a suggestion that nutrition experts often make to encourage us to eat more fruit and vegetables, but what do they really mean?.

The vitamins, minerals and antioxidants (substances that can prevent cell damage) found in plant foods are often contained in the pigments that give them their colour. Beta-carotene, which our bodies convert to vitamin A, for example, is what gives orange vegetables like carrots and butternut squash their vibrant shade. Anthocyanins are valuable antioxidants and are found in red, purple and blue pigments that colour fruit like cherries and berries.

The more colourful the range of plant-based foods we can eat, the greater the variety of nutrients we'll be taking in. In addition we know that a diverse diet is better for our gut microbes (and so for our overall physical and mental health, too). How many colours can you eat today? If you like, tick annotate the wheel opposite with the foods you eat today.

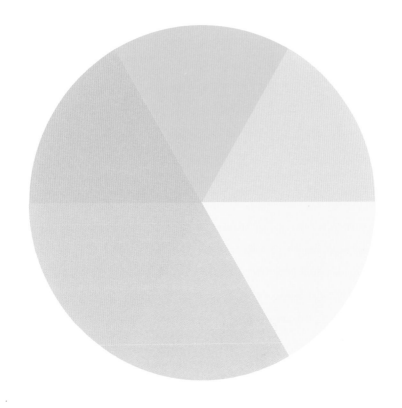

MAKE TEA – MINDFULLY

How many times do you boil the kettle and then come into the kitchen to find a stewed mug of tea with the bag still in it, or your half-drunk cup sitting cold on a shelf? Next time you go to make yourself a hot drink, do it mindfully and reclaim five minutes of calm and comfort in your day.

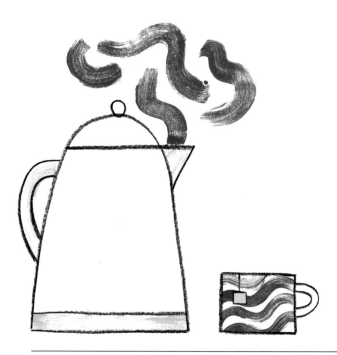

• Fill the kettle, then choose your favourite mug and teaspoon.

• Select a teabag – did you know matcha tea contains a substance called L-theanine, which studies have shown induces the same feelings of calm and alertness as meditation? And research from the British Tea Advisory Panel shows that drinking four to five cups of green or black tea a day can lower blood pressure and cholesterol, reducing the risk of heart disease and strokes.

• Boil the kettle. Listen to the noise of the water, feel the mug in your hand.

• Pour the boiled water into the mug and stir.

• Take your tea and sit quietly somewhere. Continue to be mindful as you wait for it to cool, and with each sip you take. How does it look? Smell? Taste? Feel? Sound?

COLOUR IN THIS TO FEEL NOURISHED

Spend five minutes colouring in this mandala – a circular symbol representing the universe. Choose shades and combinations that make you feel nourished and vibrant.

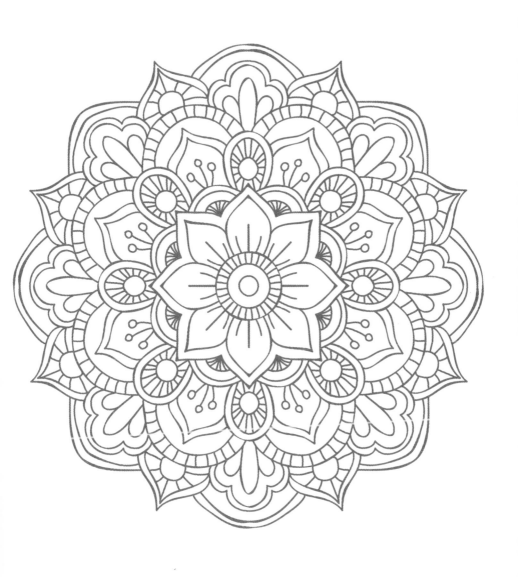

ADD FIVE MINUTES TO YOUR MEALTIMES . . .

"Nature will castigate those who don't masticate."

HORACE FLETCHER, HEALTH-FOOD ENTHUSIAST

. . . and spend it chewing your food. Good digestion begins in the mouth and chewing triggers the production of saliva, which is filled with digestive enzymes that begin breaking down your food straight away. Swallowing chunks of improperly chewed food creates a lot of extra work for the rest of your digestive system and can result in symptoms like indigestion, heartburn, bloating and the malabsorption of nutrients. At the famous Mayr health clinic in Austria, patients are given stale bread at mealtimes to remind them what's involved in chewing properly! Take smaller bites, chew until the food has lost its taste and is liquified, then swallow before putting more food in your mouth.

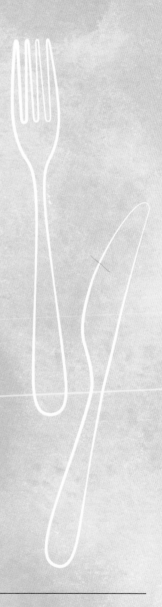

FEEL THE BEET

Beetroot isn't just for pickling. Chop the raw vegetable into matchsticks and add to salads. Or enjoy its earthy taste in a fresh, energizing, nutrient-packed juice. Beetroot works best juiced alongside carrots, apples, celery or a combination. Add 2.5cm (1in) of peeled ginger and a generous squeeze of lemon juice for an extra kick.

This vibrant vegetable is a good source of fibre, folic acid, manganese and potassium. Its purple pigment is due to betacyanin, a cancer-fighting antioxidant, and it also provides the amino acid glutamine, which plays a role in gut health. Studies show that the nitrates in beetroot may help to dilate blood vessels, reduce blood pressure and boost stamina and athletic performance. Don't discard the leaves when preparing your beetroot, either. They're a good source of vitamins A and C, calcium and iron. Lightly steam them like spinach and serve as a side dish with dinner.

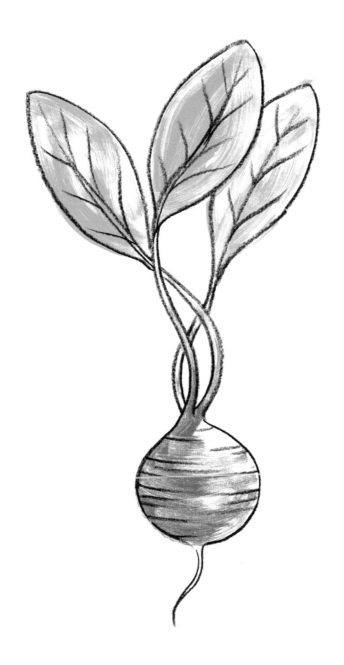

DESCRIBE A HEALTHY MEAL YOU'VE ENJOYED . . .

What made it so nourishing? How did it look, smell, feel, taste? How did it make *you* feel? Go into as much detail as you can, as if you're a top food critic describing a Michelin-starred dish.

MAKE SOME
OVERNIGHT OATS

Known as Bircher muesli, this is a low-effort way to start your day with a burst of health. Less than five minutes' preparation before bed will mean you have a delicious, filling and nutritious breakfast waiting for you by morning. And it need never be boring because, while the basic recipe remains the same, the possibilities are endless:

- Fill a single-portion jar or bowl with porridge or jumbo oats – around 60g (2oz) is a good guide.

- Top with your choice of fruit juice, natural yoghurt, kefir or nut milk: enough so that the oats are wet, but not submerged.

- Add a small handful of nuts, dried fruit or toasted seeds.

- Grate in half an apple or pear.

- If you like, add a teaspoon of chia seeds, raw cacao, macha powder or spirulina.

- Stir, cover and place in the fridge overnight.

- In the morning, top with some chopped fresh fruit and enjoy.

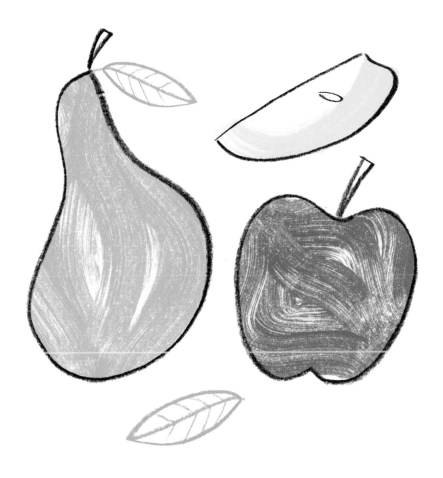

PLAN YOUR WEEK'S MEALS

It's often when we're unprepared and faced with multiple options that we make less healthy food choices: that grab-and-go meal deal from the supermarket next to your workplace; that takeaway ordered because you're home late and faced with an empty fridge. Spending a few moments planning your meals for the following week will enable you to shop accordingly, maybe even batch-cook, and resist junk-food cravings. It also takes away that 6pm "What on earth shall we have for dinner?" panic. And research proves it's associated with better dietary variety, food quality and healthier body weight.

In the space opposite, brainstorm a list of your favourite go-to meals and healthy recipes. Even if you focus just on evening meals to start with, you'll notice the benefits. Plan which meal you're going to have on each day, keeping in mind that if you make double portions, you can have leftovers for lunch or dinner for the next day or two, adding some fresh salad or vegetables.

MY HEALTHY MEALS

Monday:

Tuesday:

Wednesday:

Thursday:

Friday:

Saturday:

Sunday:

SHOPPING LIST

PURGE ONE SHELF
IN YOUR PANTRY

Choose one shelf in your kitchen store cupboard or pantry and take everything out. Go through and check the use-by dates on all the foods. Throw out anything that's out of date. Put to one side anything you don't like, won't use or have too much of – you can donate it to a food bank. Get rid of anything unhealthy that you always find too tempting: sugary snacks and highly processed foods.

Give the shelf a quick clean and put everything you're keeping back in there, making a note of any items you need to replenish or replace.

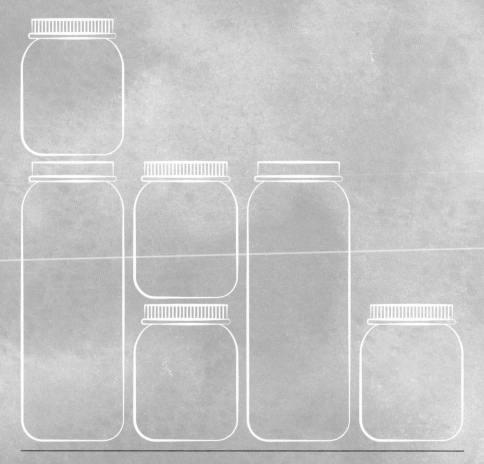

FILL UP ON FERMENTS

Fermented foods and drinks are teeming with naturally occurring probiotics – bacteria that make their way through the digestive system to the gut, where they make our microbiome (the microorganisms in the human body) more abundant and varied.

Add one of the following fermented items to your list each time you go shopping. Aim to include these probiotic foods and drinks daily, for a bacterial boost to benefit your digestion, energy levels, mood, complexion and overall wellbeing:

- Natural yoghurt
- Kefir
- Kombucha
- Miso
- Sauerkraut
- Kimchi
- Fermented tofu
- Natto
- Sourdough bread

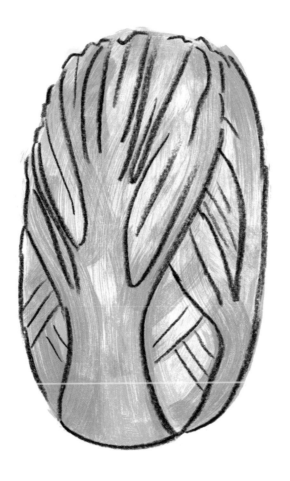

SATISFY A SWEET TOOTH, THE HEALTHY WAY

Avoid the added sugars in traditional jams and spreads by making your own chia/berry jam. It's easy, takes just five minutes and can last a week in the fridge. Enjoy it spread on toast, oatcakes, crackers, pancakes and more.

- Place a punnet of your favourite berriesin a saucepan with a splash of water. Heat gently until lightly stewed.

- Mash them with a fork, adding some cinnamon to taste, if desired.

- Stir in 1–2 tablespoons of chia seeds – these will develop a thick, jelly-like consistency.

- Add a squeeze of lemon juice and stir

- Once cooled, transfer the jam to a clean, lidded jar.

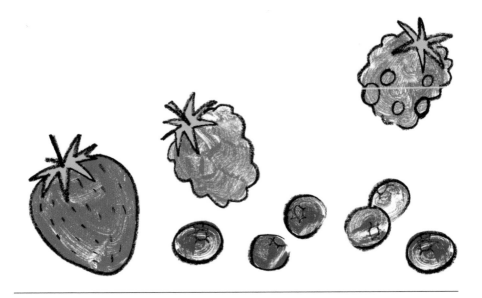

CHOOSE YOUR "EATING WINDOW"

There's increasing evidence in favour of time-restricted eating – basically, increasing your overnight fast so that you spend fewer hours of the day eating. Giving your digestive system a longer break between meals is thought to benefit your microbiome. While it's not busy digesting, a new set of gut bugs can come in and "clean up" the gut wall. Intermittent fasting has also been linked to greater longevity, lower disease risk and weight loss.

The basic premise is to consume all your day's food within a set time frame – rather than grazing from the moment you wake until you go to bed. You could start by aiming to have your meals within 12 hours, then fast for the other 12 hours. So if you have breakfast at 8am, you need to finish dinner by 8pm, then fast until 8am again – water and herbal teas are fine, though.

If that feels easy, you could try a 14:10 or 16:8 ratio. This might mean missing a meal, rather than trying to cram all three meals into a shorter timeframe. So for the 16:8 plan, you might skip breakfast and have your first meal at noon, then finish your evening meal by 8pm. Or, if you prefer to eat early, you might breakfast at 8am, then finish eating for the day by 4pm.

WHIZZ UP A SOUP

It takes just minutes to chop up some healthy ingredients, sauté them in oil, add stock to cook them and whizz up the result in a blender. But this small investment of your time could provide you with a week's worth of filling, nutritious lunches or dinners. You can pack a whole day's nutrition into one hearty bowl. Plus, there's good evidence that eating soup can aid weight loss. Eating the same ingredients in liquid form, rather than as whole foods, means your stomach takes longer to empty and you feel fuller and more satisfied for longer.

Take a look in your fridge and store cupboard and see what "leftovers soup" you could make today. Don't forget you can add grains, pulses, nuts and seeds, herbs and spices to your vegetable base, as well as meat, fish or tofu, if desired.

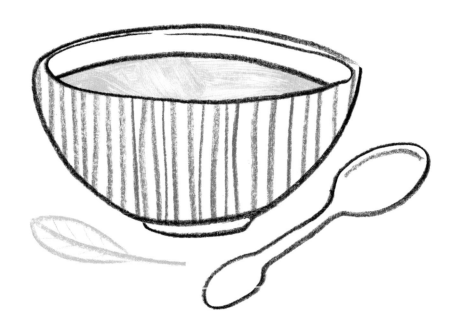

RESTORE

"The best advice is found on the pillow." **DANISH PROVERB**

You deserve to sleep well. In this chapter we'll look at everything from breathing techniques to creating a sacred space to relax in, mind tricks to switch off and what to eat, drink and do before bed to help you drift into the arms of Morpheus.

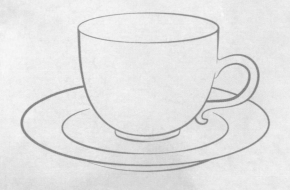

DUMP YOUR TO-DO LIST

Do you fall into bed exhausted, but find that while your body is ready to rest, your mind has other ideas? If you can't quiet the mental chatter, keep this journal and a pen on your bedside table. Before you turn out the light, spend five minutes "downloading" the contents of your whirring brain onto paper.

Instead of racing through tomorrow's to-do list in your mind, note down each item, in bullet points. Whatever comes into your head, by writing it down you can release those thoughts, let them go – at least until morning – and leave your mind to rest. Studies have shown this is an effective technique that promotes better sleep.

SEAL THE DAY

Research has shown that being positive and thankful increases happiness and self-esteem, reduces depression and can even improve sleep quality and duration. At the end of each day, take some time to focus on its positives. However hard the day may have been, you can always find optimism and gratitude. Write down:

• Three good things that have happened to you today, however small

• Three people you wish well to

•Three things you can look forward to tomorrow.

Get into the habit of doing this every evening. It doesn't have to be before bed – if you live with others, you could share your thoughts over dinner.

CLEAR YOUR BEDSIDE CLUTTER

"Have nothing in your houses that you do not know to be useful, or believe to be beautiful." **WILLIAM MORRIS**

Spend five minutes tidying and dusting your bedside table and getting rid of anything that doesn't need to be there. Turn what remains there into your sleep shrine. Collect items that make you feel peaceful or can be used in a pre-bed ritual for sleep: a book to read, a small notebook and pen, a pretty glass for water, an aromatherapy pillow spray or wrist roller, ear plugs or an eye mask, if you use either. Keep ornaments to a minimum – a photograph of a loved one or natural scene. If you believe in crystal healing, add an amethyst, rose quartz or angelite to your shrine.

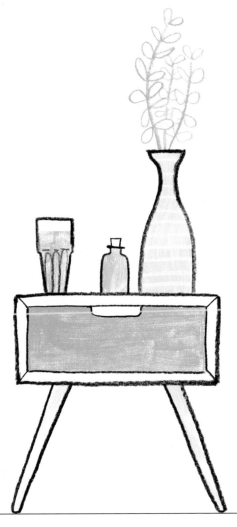

GO TO THE DARK SIDE

To sleep well, it's important to have a completely dark room. Our ancestors would have slept from dusk till dawn, with no natural or artificial light present. The body produces the hormone melatonin in response to a lack of light in the evenings, and it's this hormone that helps us to sleep and triggers all those important, restorative processes in the body. If there's too much light around, our production of melatonin – and therefore our sleep – can be compromised.

This evening, after dark, take a look at how much light is getting into your bedroom. Note down all the sources, and how you might get rid of them. If it's light from a street lamp or the moon, can you fit a blackout blind? If it's a standby LED from an electronic device, does it have to be in your room – could you swap electronic clock alarms for analogue ones and switch off other devices at the wall? Can you block light around the door, if landing- or night-lights from other rooms in the home are penetrating it? If all else fails, can you buy a comfortable eye mask? Make a blackout plan, then carry it out.

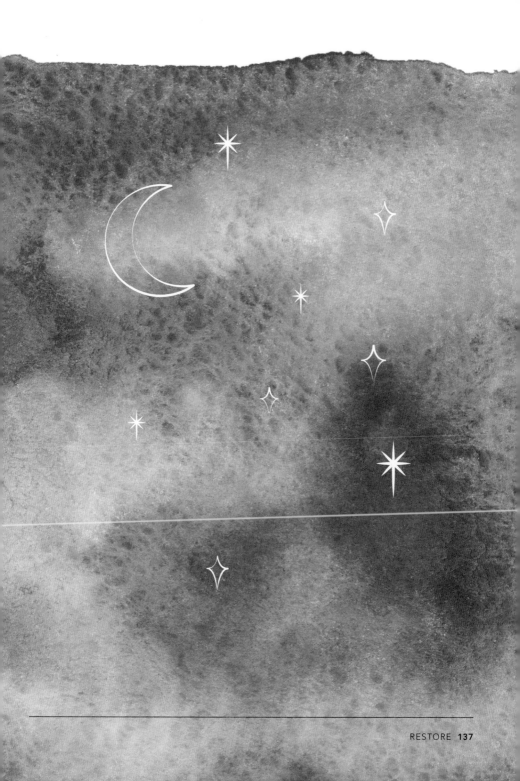

CHECK THE TEMPERATURE

Another important element of good sleep hygiene is the temperature of your bedroom. Too cold and you'll be kept awake by chilly extremities. Too warm and you'll be tossing and turning and will wake feeling groggy. Experts say the ideal room temperature is 18°C (64°F).

A useful idea is to have layers to hand, so that you can add and remove blankets, sheets or bedsocks as you need them. A source of fresh air is preferable, if it's not too cold or noisy to keep a window open. If you share a bed, look to northern Europe, where it's common to have separate duvets so that each partner can regulate their own preferred temperature.

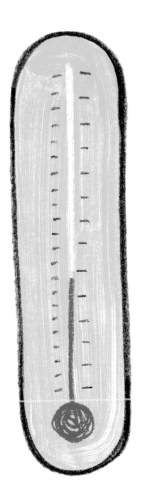

DRIFT OFF TO SLEEP WITH LEFT-NOSTRIL BREATHING

In kundalini yoga, known as "the mother of all yogas", the practice of breathing through the left nostril only is thought to be calming and soothing. It activates the relaxing part of the nervous system and so can be a valuable tool for inducing sleep.

- Sitting up straight, hold your right nostril closed with your right fingers.

- Breathe slowly and deeply, in and out, through your left nostril. As you breathe in, let your navel expand, then your ribcage. As you exhale, draw the ribcage and then the navel in toward your spine.

- Breathe like this for a few minutes, then release the right nostril and return to normal breathing as you lie down and drift off to sleep.

If you prefer and it's comfortable, you can lie on your front to perform the exercise, with your right cheek on the pillow, as this opens the left nostril to let that soothing breath in.

FLOAT, FLOAT ON . . .

You don't have to visit a flotation tank – or the Dead Sea – to harness the restorative benefits of floating. Remember how wonderful it feels to lie back in the sea and let the salt water hold you buoyant? Try to replicate that the next time you're swimming, or even in the bath. Lying on your back with your ears submerged and your eyes closed takes you into a world of sensory deprivation, which helps to relieve muscle tension and ease stress.

Being cocooned in warmth and silence seems to have a positive effect on the brain. Scientists have been studying the effects of sensory-deprivation flotation since the 1950s and have found benefits for both anxiety and depression. It's so effective that doctors in Sweden are able to prescribe flotation sessions. Add some Epsom salts or magnesium flakes to your bath to further enhance relaxation, aid muscle recovery and promote restful sleep.

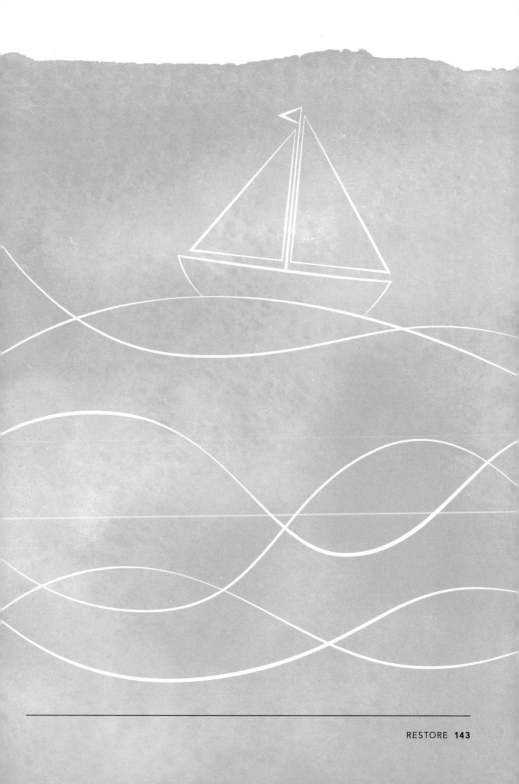

SWITCH UP YOUR EVENING DRINKS

If you struggle to nod off at night, you probably know that caffeine before bed is a bad idea. But how early should you quit the tea and coffee? Studies suggest it can take six to twelve hours for caffeine to leave your system, so it's a good idea to switch to decaffeinated or herbal hot drinks from mid-afternoon onward. Caffeine keeps us alert by blocking the brain-chemical adenosine, which makes us feel drowsy – great in the mornings or before a big meeting or long drive, but not so handy at night. Instead, choose calming, soporific infusions of herbs like valerian, lemon balm, hops and rose.

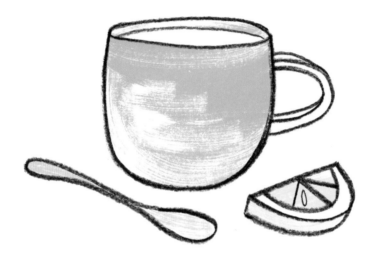

BUILD A BESPOKE
BEDTIME OIL BLEND

Essential oils can help to induce sleep safely and naturally, without any nasty side-effects. Top aromatherapist Mary Dalgleish recommends lavender, chamomile and neroli as being calming, soothing and useful for relieving anxiety, which can hinder sleep. Her favourite sedatives include vetiver, valerian, clary sage, marjoram, benzoin and bergamot, which is also uplifting.

Choose two or three of the above oils to make a blend (four to six drops in total) – go for scents that most appeal when you sniff the bottle. You can experiment each time you do this, until you find a combination you really love. Then try any of the following remedies:

• Dilute your blend in 10ml (2tsp) of carrier oil (try sweet almond or jojoba) or some milk, before adding to a warm bath before bedtime. Make sure it's not too hot, as this can stimulate rather than relax.

• Use the diluted oil blend to massage your feet before bedtime.

• Add the essential oils (undiluted) to a diffuser in your bedroom.

• Inhale them from a tissue.

• Sprinkle a few drops onto your pillow.

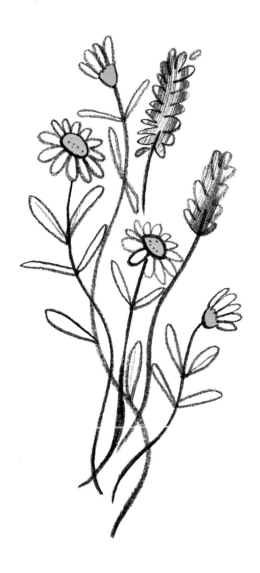

TRY THIS
WIND-DOWN
YOGA PRACTICE

Having a short yoga sequence to practise before bed can be a wonderful way to prepare for, and promote, restful sleep.

"Choose forward bends and inversions, as these calm the mind and relax the body," says yoga teacher Rebecca Oura. "Back-bends, conversely, can be too stimulating. A good, nurturing sequence could begin with Child's Pose, then move through Cat/Cow, Downward Dog and a gentle spinal twist (lying on your back, knees raised, feet on the floor, arms out at shoulder height; drop the knees to one side, head to the other, and vice versa). Finish by lying on your back, a folded blanket under your hips, and raise your legs at a right angle to your body. You can either rest them against a wall, or use a belt or scarf around your feet. This position stimulates the pineal gland, increasing that all-important evening melatonin production."

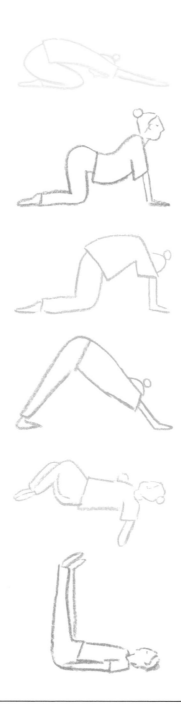

SLASH YOUR SCREEN TIME

Modern life means that we spend a great deal of time looking at screens: from our work computers to home laptops, smartphones to tablets, games consoles to TVs. In the evening this habit can be particularly damaging to sleep. The type of blue light these screens emit is found in nature mainly in the mornings and early afternoons. If we're exposed to it in the evenings, it suppresses the body's natural production of melatonin. This helps govern our circadian rhythms and signals to the brain that we're ready for sleep.

If you struggle to get to sleep, spend five minutes looking into measures to reduce your blue-light exposure of an evening. Most smartphones can be switched onto night-time mode, which is a warmer light source. There are also apps to do this for phones and tablets. Or you can buy screen covers or blue-light cancelling glasses. Television may not be as detrimental, as we tend to sit further from the screen. But the best way to prepare body and mind for sleep is to switch off all screens and devices for a couple of hours before bed.

PICK UP A GOOD BOOK

"A book is a dream that you hold in your hand."

NEIL GAIMAN, WRITER

Bedtime stories aren't just for children. The tradition of reading before sleep has been well studied and there's plenty of evidence that it helps us drift off. A book isn't simply a distraction – experts say that by actively engaging your imagination, reading helps put your mind into an altered state of consciousness, preparing it for sleep. Studies have shown that just six minutes of reading can reduce stress levels by 68 per cent.

Bookworms can also sleep more soundly knowing that the habit is boosting their cognitive function, memory and empathy. It doesn't matter what genre of book, so long as you find it fully absorbing.

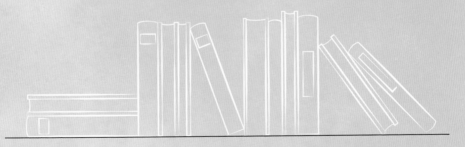

MAKE LIKE THE MILITARY

The following is a technique reputedly designed by the US military to help its pilots get to sleep in just two minutes. The method boasts a 96 per cent success rate with six weeks of practice.

- Relax your face, including your tongue, jaw and the muscles around your eyes.

- Drop your shoulders as low as they can go. Then relax your upper and lower arm on one side, and then the other.

- Breathe out and relax your chest.

- Relax your legs, from the thighs to the calves.

- When your mind is clear, picture one of the following images: lying in a canoe on a calm lake with nothing but blue sky above you; being snuggled in a black velvet hammock in a pitch-black room, saying, "Don't think, don't think, don't think" over and over again.

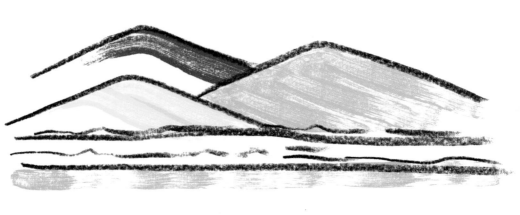

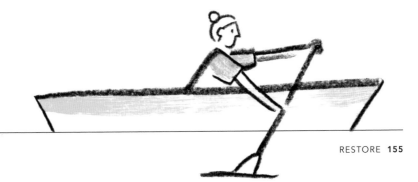

DREAM, BABY, DREAM

"In all chaos there is a cosmos, in all disorder a secret order."

CARL JUNG, PSYCHIATRIST AND PSYCHOANALYST

The space on the oppsoite page is for you to record everything you can remember about what you dreamed last night. Sometimes it's hard to recall later in the day, so if nothing comes to mind, keep this journal by your bed and save this exercise for tomorrow, on waking. Or you can start by writing about a past or recurring dream that sticks in your mind.

A dream journal is more than a personal treasure. Psychologists believe it's a valuable tool for learning more about yourself. By noting down your dreams on a regular basis, you're able to look at themes and patterns that occur over time. Try to include as much detail as you can, particularly about how you were feeling in the dream, as well as what was happening. When you've finished, give your dream a title.

HOW DID YOU SLEEP?

*"There is a time for many words,
and there is also a time for sleep."*

HOMER, EPIC POET

Use the space opposite to record as much as you can about how you slept last night.
Include as much practical and emotional detail as possible. Depending on whether
you had a good or poor night's sleep, these details can, over time, help to build a
picture of what works or doesn't work for you. Repeat this exercise whenever you
remember in the mornings, to help you perfect your personal sleep recipe.

- Where did you sleep?
- What did you eat/drink/do in the hours leading up to bedtime?
- What time did you get into bed?
- What did you wear?
- Did your bedroom feel comfortable?
- Did you perform any pre-sleep rituals (such as aromatherapy, yoga, relaxation techniques, reading)?
- How soon do you think you fell asleep?
- Did you wake during the night?
- If so, what did you do?
- What time did you wake up and get up?
- How did you feel when you woke?

ACKNOWLEDGMENTS

Picture credits: Artulina1/iStock 39, 160; Visnezh/Dreamstime 107.

Acknowledgments

p.10, Copyright © Ralph Waldo Emerson 1850; p.26, Copyright © Miriam Akhtar, The Little Book of Happiness 2019; p. 42, Copyright © Gary Keller, The One Thing 2013; p. 46, Copyright © Metta Sutta; p. 62, Copyright © Dr Seuss, You're Only Old Once 1986; p.74, Copyright © Martin Gibala, The One Minute Workout 2017; p.92, Copyright © Martha Graham, US choreographer and dancer; p.94, Copyright © Jean Anthelme Brillat-Savarin, The Physiology of Taste 1825; p.108, Copyright © Horace Fletcher, The A.B-Z of Our Own Nutrition (1903); p.134, Copyright © William Morris, "The Beauty of Life" 1880; p.148, Copyright © Rebecca Oura, Yoga Teacher; p.152, Copyright © Neil Gaiman, Author ; p.156, © Carl Jung, The Archetypes and the Collective Unconscious 1959; p.158, © Homer, The Odyssey

2	5	6	8	3	7	1	4	9
7	1	9	4	2	5	8	3	6
8	4	3	6	1	9	2	5	7
4	6	7	1	5	8	9	2	3
3	9	2	7	6	4	5	1	8
5	8	1	3	9	2	6	7	4
1	7	8	2	4	6	3	9	5
6	3	5	9	7	1	4	8	2
9	2	4	5	8	3	7	6	1

Contributor: Hannah Ebelthite
Consultant Publisher: Kate Adams
Editorial Assistant: Cara Armstrong
Copyeditor: Mandy Greenfield
Senior Designer: Geoff Fennell
Designer & Illustrator: Ella Mclean
Deputy Picture Manager: Jen Veall
Picture Research Manager: Giulia Hetherington
Production Manager: Lisa Pinnell